M000035266

TANSY BRIGGS, DACM

# The Key to
# INFANT NUTRITION

Using The Warm Digestion Principle
to Guide Your Baby from Breast or
Bottle to Eating Food

Publishing Services provided by Paper Raven Books

Printed in the United States of America

First Printing, 2020

Paperback ISBN= 978-1-7340561-2-9
Hardback ISBN= 978-1-7340561-3-6

# Dedication

*This book is dedicated to all the parents and babies I have come to know through my practice who have been willing to try my advice. Without them, I never would have been motivated to put the original guide together many years ago, then tweak and improve it over the years, and now put it in a more readable, expanded and user-friendly form! May this book continue to help parents and babies for many more years to come.*

# TABLE OF CONTENTS

# INTRODUCTION

. . . . . . . . . . . . . . . . . . . .

*Establishing a warm*
*digestion in your baby*
*and why it's important*

. . . . . . . . . . . . . . . . . . . .

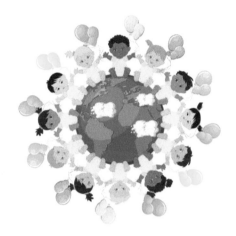

Whether you're having your first baby or third, you know the anxiety of wanting to "get it right" when raising your child. You worry about your baby crying for hours with colic, about child obesity or malnourishment, chronic illnesses or allergies, whether you will or can breastfeed, bad reactions to vaccinations, and so many other considerations that your head begins to spin. As it turns out, you're not wrong to worry. Studies have shown that the first 1,000 days of life are a crucial time for nutrition that can have lasting health effects for the rest of one's life.

*As shown by an analysis of evidence-based interventions, a focus on improvements in nutrition during pregnancy and linear growth of a child in the first two years of life could lead to substantial reductions in stunting and improvements in survival. These improvements, which have been used effectively to scale up nutrition activities, form the basis for the emphasis on the first 1,000 days of life. (Bhutta, 2013)*

How about a common sense approach that can be incorporated into any lifestyle, cultural food approach and formula, or breastfeeding routine?

We'll talk more in depth about what warm digestion is, but, essentially, a body that is experiencing warm digestion processes food easily, absorbs nutrients from foods efficiently, and provides energy to all parts of the body. If you get warm digestion right, many other health concerns are immediately relieved and the body is healthy and resilient.

What you will learn in this guide:

1. How warm digestion can affect breastfeeding and heal your body postpartum.

2. What you need to know to keep your baby's digestion warm if feeding your baby formula.

3. How to transition your baby to solid foods, keeping to the warm digestion principles, and why it's important.

4. How the warm digestion principles can positively affect conditions such as colic, reflux, bloating, irregular bowel movements (constipation or diarrhea), teething, sleeping, growth and development, disposition, illnesses, reactions to vaccinations, immunity, and life transitions.

5. How the warm digestion principles can set your baby up for a lifetime of healthy digestion and resilient health.

# WHAT IS THE WARM DIGESTION PRINCIPLE?

. . . . . . . . . . . . . . . . . . . .

*What Chinese Medicine
has taught us about how
to keep our digestion
healthy*

. . . . . . . . . . . . . . . . . . . .

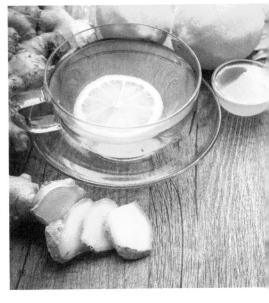

Chinese Medicine uses an analogy for how our bodies process food. Think of your digestive system as a soup pot that needs to reach a certain temperature to begin to "cook" your food.

All foods, herbs, and spices are categorized and have a temperature, ranging from cold to hot. Cooking, as well as certain ways of preparing food, such as adding spices, can help change the temperature qualities of some foods. For example, iced water is cold, but you can warm water to a neutral room temperature or you can boil it to make it hot. The more cool foods and drinks you have, the harder your digestive system must work in order to "heat" the food to properly digest.

A "warm" digestive system will process the food quickly, easily, and efficiently, giving us energy and resilient health. A "cool" digestive system can be sluggish or painful, which we may experience as gas, bloating, cramps, constipation, reflux, phlegm, and frequent illnesses.

Chinese Medicine is about seeking balance in all areas of life, including food and digestion. Having a balance of temperatures, flavors, and foods greatly enhances health. Chinese Medicine has shown that many of our pains and illnesses dissipate when we warm up our digestion. Using the principles of warm digestion, I have treated adults and children since 2002, and I have seen how directly and immediately a warm digestion can clear up chronic illnesses, pains, allergies, and even emotional issues. Using the principles of warm and cool digestion gives us a wonderful tool to fine-tune known nutritional guidelines and specific diet plans.

## ■ WHAT FOODS AFFECT THE TEMPERATURE OF OUR DIGESTION?

I give a thorough explanation of exactly what foods to eat for warm digestion, and why, in my book, *The Key to a Healthy Digestion: How to Eat Warm and Cold Foods to Improve Your Health*, but I'd like to give you a brief description here.

Generally:

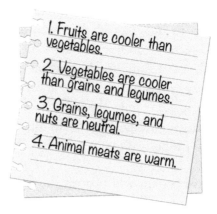

1. Fruits are cooler than vegetables.
2. Vegetables are cooler than grains and legumes.
3. Grains, legumes, and nuts are neutral.
4. Animal meats are warm.

Within each category, though, there is a range of temperatures. Grains, legumes, and nuts are neutral; soy is cooler than rice; and rice is cooler than oats. Let's go through examples of the temperatures of foods within each category.

# FRUITS:

| | |
|---|---|
| **Cold** | banana, blueberry, cantaloupe, cranberry, grapefruit, kiwi, mango, mulberry, persimmon, plum, rhubarb, tomato, watermelon |
| **Cool** | apple, avocado, blackcurrant, coconut, orange, pear, prune, tangerine |
| **Neutral** | apricot, lemon, loquat, papaya, peach, pomegranate, tangerine |
| **Warm** | blackberry, cherry, date, fig, grape, kumquat, longan, lychee, quince, raspberry, strawberry |
| **Hot** | pineapple |

# VEGETABLES:

| | |
|---|---|
| **Cold** | asparagus, Chinese cabbage, dandelion leaf, seaweed, snow pea, water chestnut, white mushroom |
| **Cool** | alfalfa sprout, artichoke, bamboo shoot, bok choy, broccoli, carrot, cauliflower, celery, corn, cucumber, daikon radish, eggplant, endive, mushroom, potato, romaine lettuce, spinach, swiss chard, tomato, turnip, zucchini |
| **Neutral** | beet, cabbage, carrot, collard greens, lettuce, olive, pea, pumpkin, shiitake mushroom, yam |

| | |
|---|---|
| **Warm** | bell pepper, chive, fennel, green bean, kale, leek, mustard greens, onion, oyster mushroom, parsley, parsnip, scallion, squash, sweet potato, watercress |
| **Hot** | garlic, green onion |

## GRAINS, LEGUMES, AND NUTS:

| | |
|---|---|
| **Cold** | wheat germ |
| **Cool** | amaranth, barley, buckwheat, lima bean, millet, mung bean, soybean, wheat, wild rice |
| **Neutral** | almond, brown rice, chickpea, corn, flax, hazelnut, peanut, pistachio, pumpkin, sunflower seed, white rice |
| **Warm** | black bean, chestnut, oats, pine nut, quinoa, safflower, sesame seed, spelt, walnut |

## ANIMAL PRODUCTS:

| | |
|---|---|
| **Cold** | clam, crab, octopus |
| **Cool** | eggs, pork, duck |
| **Neutral** | abalone, rabbit, cheese, chicken, duck, goose, herring, mackerel, milk, oyster, salmon, sardine, shark, tuna |

| Warm | anchovy, beef, butter, chicken, eel, fresh water fish, goat, ham, lobster, mussel, sheep, sheep's milk, shrimp, turkey, venison |
|---|---|
| Hot | lamb, trout |

## ■ SPICES AND OILS:

| Cold | salt, white pepper |
|---|---|
| Cool | cilantro leaf, marjoram, mint, peppermint, sesame oil, tamarind |
| Neutral | coriander, licorice, olive oil, peanut oil, saffron |
| Warm | anise, basil, bay leaf, carob, caraway, clove, coriander, cumin, dill seed, fennel, fenugreek, fresh ginger, jasmine, nutmeg, oregano, rosemary, sage, spearmint, thyme |
| Hot | black pepper, cayenne pepper, chili pepper, cinnamon, garlic, dry ginger, horseradish, mustard, wasabi |

Within each category, though, there is a range of temperatures. If you're trying to warm up your digestion, you will want to avoid fruits and raw vegetables for the most part. This is by no means an exhaustive list! You can take these lists and experiment and even add your own foods as well. At the end of the day, you are the best judge of your body.

# HOW DOES WARM DIGESTION APPLY TO INFANTS AND CHILDREN?

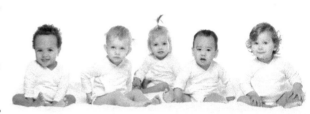

The baby develops inside the mother's womb at her body temperature, and when the baby is out in the world, he drinks his mother's milk, also at body temperature. However, if you do a quick Internet search, more often than not, many sources will say it doesn't matter if the baby's milk is served cold, at room temperature, or warm. There is a consensus that microwaves are problematic in heating milk, as it can heat unevenly and form hot spots.

We know that, according to pediatric guidelines, a baby's digestion is working optimally if she's producing a certain number of wet and dirty diapers according to age every 24 hours. (Mohrbacher, 2010-2019)

But what do we do when our baby suddenly becomes irritable, gassy, or colicky? And what do we do when our baby is ready for nutrition, beyond breast milk or formula?

Let's go into the next chapter to talk about how to make sure your baby's digestion is staying warm, resilient, and healthy.[1]

1 *General Guidelines here are based on optimal health; this does not take into account individual philosophies or health conditions.*

# POSTPARTUM NUTRITION

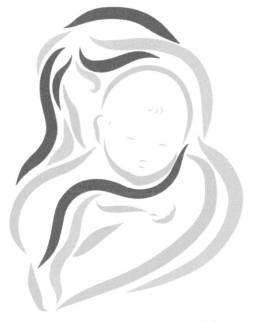

*Help your body
heal and produce
nourishing milk
using the warm
digestion principle*

It's very important to eat warming and nourishing foods, especially for the first three months after giving birth and then throughout breastfeeding. This will help your body heal, support breastfeeding, and help your baby have a healthy digestion, reducing the possibility of colic and other digestive upsets. This concept is expanded in the *Key To Postpartum Healing* book. However, we will summarize here as well.

If your digestion is cool or cold, your ability to properly digest food is weakened. You may physically feel the effects of a cool digestion as slow healing after childbirth, slowness to lose the pregnancy weight, irregular digestion, and fatigue. If you are breastfeeding, this may also affect the digestion of your newborn, which manifests as gas, bloating, colic, and reflux (or frequent spitting up).

## ■ 8 WAYS YOU CAN HAVE WARM DIGESTION ON A DAILY BASIS

**1.** Start your day with a warm, cooked breakfast. Include warming proteins with your breakfast.

**2.** Drink only warm or room temperature beverages.

**3.** Eat lots of soups and stews, such as bone broth, miso soup, chicken soup, and beef stew.

**4.** Avoid eating leftovers right out of the refrigerator without warming.

**5.** Avoid all raw vegetables until four months after giving birth, then only eat them sparingly.

**6.** When eating dairy, choose drier and harder cheeses (less damp and cooling), and plain or neutral flavors of yogurt. For example, you can warm up yogurt (considered cool and damp) by adding cinnamon, which is a warming spice.

**7.** Avoid all fruits until month two after giving birth and then only more warming and/or in season fruits or cooked fruits until month four. Then, if you and baby are both digesting well, you can experiment a bit more.

**8.** Avoiding most foods on the inflammatory list (listed later in this chapter) until month four after giving birth can be helpful, especially if baby is more reactive digestively.

**Vegetables during postpartum.** You can eat from the entire list of vegetables, but you should cook the foods first to keep to the warming principle. However, be sparing with nightshade vegetables (such as bell peppers, tomatoes, and eggplants) as they are considered more inflammatory and can affect your breast milk and upset your baby's digestion.

**Other nutrient concerns while breastfeeding.** Specific estimates are based on the Recommended Dietary Allowance, RDA, and other studies taking into account varied milk output, different diets, ethnic background, quality of food, and age of the mother. (Institute of Medicine (US) Committee on Nutritional Status During Pregnancy and Lactation., 1991):

1. Eat 60 to 65 g of warming protein daily.

2. Drink at least 8 to 12 oz of balanced electrolytes daily (suggested recipes below).

3. Consume good oils, such as a DHA supplement or 1 tsp of real olive oil daily.

4. When you do use salt, use good salt, such as sea salt or mined salt.

5. Drink plenty of warm teas and drinks. Avoid cold or iced drinks altogether.

6. Incorporate bone minerals through bone broth soups. Bone mineral supplements may also be considered to support bone health.

7. Reduce inflammatory foods. This is always important, but particularly during postpartum and breastfeeding.

**8.** Avoiding most foods on the inflammatory list (listed later in this chapter) until month four after giving birth can be helpful, especially if baby is more reactive digestively.

## ELECTROLYTES RECIPES

**1.** There are numerous retail products available, but try to avoid ones high in sugar.

**2.** Consider adding a powdered electrolyte mix to water that contains less sugar. There are many good options you can buy these days.

**3.** Make your own: 1 tablespoon of lemon juice with 1/2 teaspoon of a sweetener (like honey or real raw sugar) and a generous pinch of sea or unrefined salt in 8 ounces of water.

## BONE BROTH SOUP

Bone broth soup is very nourishing after childbirth and gives needed nutrients for healing and breastfeeding support. You can make it in advance and freeze it. Bone broth can then be eaten by itself or as a stock to make other soups. There are a lot of great recipes on the Internet and in cookbooks. You can also purchase organic bone broth from many grocery stores.

## INFLAMMATORY FOODS THAT MAY BE AFFECTING YOUR BREAST MILK

As much as keeping a warm digestion is important, some foods fall into an inflammatory category because they are hot or produce heat toxins in the body. If you are not sensitive to inflammation, you may have less trouble with these foods. But if you tend to have food sensitivities, you may have more severe reactions, or it can pass on to your baby while breastfeeding.

Some foods may cause physical inflammation in your digestive system, which is disruptive to a healthy digestive process. This, in turn, may affect your breast milk and cause your baby's digestion to be very reactive, which you may notice as gas, bloating, colic, or reflux (or frequent spitting up).

Below is a list of the common inflammatory food groups, and then some examples of how you can apply the warm digestion concept (where appropriate) to reduce the effect of inflammatory foods in your diet. Perhaps you don't need to completely eliminate these foods during the postpartum period or during breastfeeding. As your baby grows, their digestion will begin to mature, and foods that may have affected them more in the first month may not affect them as much by the fourth month, and so on.

**Gluten.** This includes wheat, rye, oats, and barley, which are commonly found in breads, pasta, and other products made with refined flour, and is a very common allergy and inflammatory substance. You can react to gluten from a true autoimmune reaction (celiac disease) to having sensitivity or an allergy to gluten where the reason is often unknown.

*A way to make it better by using the Warm Digestion Concept:* Sprouted grains, such as bread made from sprouted wheat, can reduce inflammation and sensitivity in the digestion.

**Alcohol, caffeine, soda, and fruit juice.** Both alcohol and caffeine can affect the functioning of the liver, kidneys, and blood sugar regulation systems, and have other long-term health and inflammation repercussions.

*A way to make it better by using the Warm Digestion Concept:* Studies have shown the benefits of moderate use of certain types of alcohol. Red wine, for instance, is warming and is used in preparations of certain Chinese herb formulas to reduce pain and provide other health benefits. For postpartum patients, there is a formula where you cook the herbs in sake (rice wine) and drink this formula for the first month after childbirth. Traditional Chinese Medicine considers even water too cooling for this time of a woman's life.

Although not necessarily inflammation causing, caffeine acts as a diuretic, as well as a stimulant, and can reduce your breast milk volume or affect your baby.

Soda (especially diet) and processed fruit drinks that are high in simple, refined, or synthetic sugars are hard on the mechanisms that regulate your blood sugar levels. High intakes of sugars, especially synthetic sugars, have been associated with inflammation.

**Certain meats.** Pork, cold cuts, bacon, hot dogs, canned meats, sausage, and shellfish, as well as meats that are not organic or naturally raised and processed, can be high in hormones, antibiotics, and other undesired ingredients utilized during processing.

*A way to make it better by using the Warm Digestion Concept:* Eat natural forms of meats without nitrates or additives.

**Corn, tomato sauce, and nightshade vegetables.** These commonly cause inflammation and allergic responses.

*A way to make it better by using the Warm Digestion Concept:* Eat more heritage strains, grown without pesticides, and eat them when they're in season.

**Eggs and dairy.** This includes all milk, cheese, butter, and yogurt because they produce dampness and phlegm in the body.

*A way to make it better by using the Warm Digestion Concept:* Eat farm fresh eggs; harder, drier cheeses; and hormone-free milk, yogurt, and butter.

**Citrus fruits, juices, and strawberries.** These are common allergens and/or phlegm producers. They also produce a cooling effect to the digestion and may adversely affect blood sugar regulation.

**Foods high in saturated fats and refined oils.** Examples are peanuts, margarine, and shortening. Processing these foods places an extra burden on the digestive system.

*A way to make it better by using the Warm Digestion Concept:* Less processed, good oils and fats have true health benefits in the body's systems.

# HOW WARM DIGESTION CAN POSITIVELY AFFECT YOUR BABY'S HEALTH

*In Chinese Medicine pediatrics, there is a concept called "changing and steaming syndromes."*

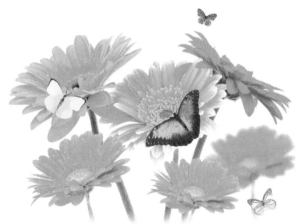

Every three to six months, from birth to age two, your baby will experience significant changes in digestion and physiology. Just as often as you have to size up your baby's clothes, you'll also see your baby going through a "changing syndrome," which shows up as a difference in appetite, change in moods, physical discomfort, changes in sleep cycles, and illnesses that may be more phlegmy, such as a noticeable runny nose.

At the same time, your baby can go through a "steaming syndrome," which you'll see as a fever, red cheeks, loss of appetite, runny stools, and even vomiting, pain, or ear infections, especially if baby's molars are coming in.

Once the changing and steaming cycles have passed, there is usually a jump in development relating to motor development or physical features, as well as a jump in brain, cognitive, or bone growth development.

> The strength of baby's digestion can directly determine how well baby will handle these cycles, as well as how baby handles vaccinations, exposure to colds and flus, seasonal changes, and even group childcare and stressful environments.

In fact, your baby's nutrition may even have an impact on emotions and sleep. Think you have a fussy, irritable, or even colicky baby on your hands? You may just have a baby with a digestive issue. Here's a conversation I had with a patient recently about her six-month-old baby:

Me: What is the most frustrating thing you are struggling with on a daily basis?

Mom: His fussiness. He can be happy one minute and unhappy the next, especially in the late afternoon or evening.

Me: What is the most bothersome daily struggle, problem, or issue?

Mom: Bedtime and nap time.

Me: How is this impacting your day? How does this make you feel?

Mom: I dread this time of day. I feel exhausted after the routine of trying to put him down, watching him on the monitor, trying to feed him, trying to calm him. There has to be an easier way!

Me: What do you wish would be different?

Mom: I wish I had more energy at the end of the day to play with him, and I wish he wasn't fussy. I'm not naturally a "baby *person" and when I'm tired, it's very hard for me to enjoy my time with him. As he gets older, it is easier because he is more interactive with play, but it is still hard to be "on," particularly during the week, and this kiddo needs that or else he becomes a fuss-muss.*

Me: If we could change one thing, what would that look like?

*Mom: A happy baby that is able to play on his own (on occasion) without becoming upset, and go down for bed and nap times easily.*

This doesn't sound very related to diet, does it? As it turns out, his digestion was not working very well. He was prone to constipation, distention, and digestive upset. He also had a chronic, lingering runny nose.

By simply adjusting what he was eating and how frequently, we were able to help him take better naps, sleep more at night, and clear up his phlegm. Overall, he became a healthier and less fussy baby. Mom was less exhausted, had the knowledge she needed to address future issues, and felt supported. Understanding the role of digestion and how to fix it helps to give a path to resolution for a lot of health issues as your baby grows.

When should we start making sure our bodies are receiving the right nutrition? From day one.

> Imagine if you could prevent prolonged illnesses, emotional upsets, and behavioral problems, just from ensuring that your child's digestive system is getting exactly the foods it needs, at the right stage of development.

I know that following nutritional guidelines can be challenging, especially on a day-to-day basis. Although these guidelines are designed to be "ideal," know that even tiny adjustments to your baby's nutrition can have profound effects on their health now and your child's overall health as she grows up. The more intentional we are about our children's eating, from the very beginning, the more we make it possible for our children to live happier, healthier lives.

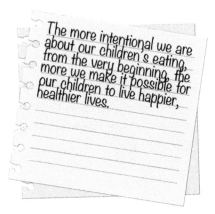

The more intentional we are about our children's eating, from the very beginning, the more we make it possible for our children to live happier, healthier lives.

# BABY'S FIRST YEAR

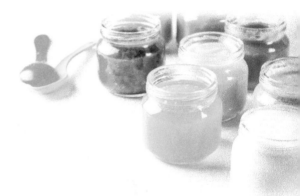

*Transitioning from breast milk or formula to solid foods*

Generally, for the first four to six months, your baby's nutrition comes exclusively from breast milk or formula. Once you begin to transition your baby to solid foods, you can slowly decrease your baby's breast milk or formula. Generally, a baby who is transitioning to solids and is between 8 and 12 months old needs about 750 to 900 calories per day with about 400 to 500 of those in the form of breast milk or formula. (American Academy of Pediatrics, 2015) Gradually, baby will increase the amount of solids he consumes so that by 18 months, about 25% of his nutrition will come from breast milk, or formula, and by 24 months, he should no longer need breast milk or formula from a nutritional perspective.

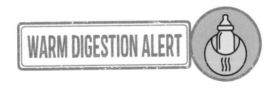

## WARM DIGESTION ALERT

### A NOTE ABOUT FORMULA AND BOTTLE FEEDING

Between you and your pediatrician, you can choose a good formula to feed your baby. Warm digestion principles recommend to always give your baby the formula at your baby's body temperature. If it is not possible to warm the formula, at least give it at room temperature and never cold. It is easier to overfeed with formula, so be sure to follow directions accordingly. Overfeeding symptoms can be: excessive spitting up and bloating with discomfort. Here's an example of how this principle played out with one of my patients: She brought her new baby in because she had colic and they were exhausted. After a few questions, I discovered they thought they were doing the right thing by giving her cold to chilled formula by adding cold water and/or premixing and keeping it refrigerated.

*"After Emma's appointment for colic and your suggestion to give her warm formula made her a new baby. Emma never had a colic fit again."*
—D. K., mother

## ■ AROUND AGE 4 TO 6 MONTHS

Around the age of 4 to 6 months, your baby will begin to show an interest for solid foods. Once baby shows an interest and is strong enough to sit up (even if she has to be supported by a pillow or towel), you can begin to introduce solid foods. It's important at this stage to go with interest as the transition to solid foods will generally go better.

## ■ START WITH CEREAL

Start with baby cereal mixed with breast milk or formula, until it reaches a runny consistency that would drip off the end of a baby spoon. Rice cereal is best, but if baby is prone to constipation, then using oatmeal cereal can relieve this issue. Try to avoid wheat-based cereals until 12 months.

Introduce solid foods as close to baby's normal schedule as possible. If your baby would normally want a large feeding around breakfast time, maybe between 6AM and 8AM, offer an ounce or two from breast or bottle (to curb intense hunger but not enough to fully satisfy), and then offer a few spoonfuls of cereal.

Offer spoonfuls of cereal again around mid-day and early evening. Continue this rhythm for a week or so before introducing other foods.

## ■ ADDING VEGGIES AND FRUITS

If your baby seems to be content after feedings and has regular wet and dirty diapers, begin adding new solid foods so that your baby can experiment with different tastes. This is an exciting time for baby! He won't love every food, at first, and he may spit many of them out, but remember that baby may need to try a food five or even ten times before he starts to enjoy it.

Introduce one new food at a time, maybe one per day. Try these options first:

1. Yellow squash

2. Peas

3. Green beans

4. Sweet potato/yams

5. Apple

6. Banana

7. Prune (especially beneficial if baby is constipated)

When choosing veggies, try to focus on low starch vegetables (examples of higher starch are potatoes and corn).

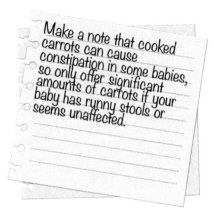

Make a note that cooked carrots can cause constipation in some babies, so only offer significant amounts of carrots if your baby has runny stools or seems unaffected.

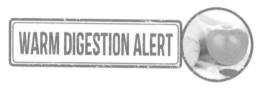

**WARM DIGESTION ALERT**

## ONLY OFFER FRUIT THREE OR FOUR TIMES A WEEK (TOTAL!)

Until your baby is at least 9 months old, or even 12 months old. **Do not offer more than one serving of fruit per day—this is a very important warm digestion consideration.** A lot of modern baby information will suggest that you feed your baby bananas and apples for nearly every feeding, but this has two problems:

**1.** Fruit cools and slows digestion, which may cause colic pains, decreased appetite, and more pain during teething.

**2.** Fruit is high in natural sugar, so too much may affect blood sugar regulation, and can cause baby to crave sweet-tasting foods, making it less likely that your baby will want to eat vegetables and proteins. It can also lead to larger fluctuations in blood sugar, which may cause irritability, more significant mood swings and can make illness, growth, and development cycles more difficult.

All cereals, veggies, and fruits should be plain (nothing added), pureed, and pure. When you are buying food in the store, look for strained, natural, and/or organic baby food.

## ▪ HOW TO COOK BABY'S FOOD

Foods that are already room temperature (like banana), you can serve without cooking, but most foods you'll need to cook to create a mushy texture and then allow to cool to room temperature.

**Steaming.** You can retain the most amount of nutrients by steaming vegetables. The vegetables should be steamed to softness, i.e., you can easily stick a fork through it. Then, it can be pureed in a blender or food processor.

**Boiling.** When vegetables sit in water and reach a boiling point, many of their nutrients pass out of the vegetable and into the water. Rather than boiling the vegetables directly in the water, try placing diced vegetables in glass containers and set the container in boiling water.

**Microwaving.** Cook the food in a glass container, not plastic, as studies have shown that certain compounds get released into the food when heated—such as pseudo hormones (chemicals that act like hormones), which can disrupt the endocrine system. (Harvard Medical School, 2017) Also, be aware that microwaves cook food faster and tend to heat the center more than the periphery, so be sure to stir the food well before serving to baby.

The younger your baby is, the smoother the puree should be. As baby gets older, you can reduce cooking and pureeing times a bit to add in more texture. Imagine small, soft chunks inside a puree, and slowly increase how "chunky" the food is, until you can just dice soft foods.

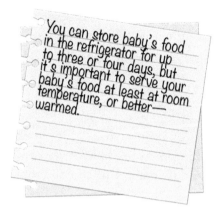

You can store baby's food in the refrigerator for up to three or four days, but it's important to serve your baby's food at least at room temperature, or better— warmed.

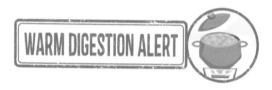

## KEEPING YOUR BABY'S DIGESTION WARM

Think of your baby's tummy as a pot of soup; it has to warm up to body temperature to start digesting (cooking). If you give your baby cold food, its immature digestion has to work that much harder, taking energy away from growth and a strong immunity. Teething and developmental growth might be more difficult or painful as a result. Thus, try to avoid raw food altogether for now.

According to the warm digestion principles, fruit is most appropriate in warm weather. Particularly during the cool months, focus on veggie and protein purees, and when the seasonal temperatures rise in the spring and summer, offer your baby fruit, but no more than once per day.

Begin to introduce sips of water during this time. You may also give diluted chamomile tea (lukewarm) as a digestive and calmative.

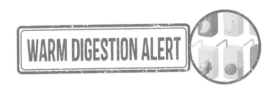

## TRY TO AVOID JUICE UNTIL 12 MONTHS

I know this sounds hard, but it is very important. Even the American Academy of Pediatrics is coming around to my way of thinking when they released new guidelines for fruit juice (although, I am not sure for the same reason as they cite juice takes away from other nutrition they need). They recommend avoiding giving juice to babies in the first year of life. (American Academy of Pediatrics, 2017)

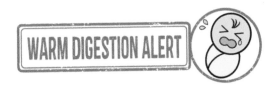

## IF YOUR BABY HAS DIGESTIVE UPSET

Slow down the introduction of solids and breastfeed or formula feed more until it clears—but don't give up! It takes time, and trying again and again, to make the transition to food. Never force feed your baby and only let him eat small amounts of solids at one time to get the idea of eating—you will avoid a lot of digestive upset this way.

## ■ AT AGE 9 MONTHS

You can begin to give teething biscuits (non-wheat preferred) at about 9 months or when your baby is really teething. Try to avoid frozen teething toys or remedies; they will seem like they help but will end up exacerbating the pain. A wet washcloth for chewing is an alternative. Consider consulting with a pediatric Chinese

Medicine practitioner or an integrative medicine pediatrician for teething and developmental pain remedies.

By this age, your baby should be consistently eating solids and trying new foods.

## ■ AT AGE 12 MONTHS

As your baby has her first birthday, breast or formula milk will be about 50% of her diet. She will be eating two to three meals of solid food per day and drinking sips of water with her meals.

*Try this schedule:*

1. Morning breakfast: solid food

2. Mid-morning snack: breast milk or formula

3. Lunch: solid food

4. Mid-afternoon snack: breast milk or formula

5. Dinner: solid food

6. Before bed: breast milk or formula

## ■ EXPAND BABY'S FOOD GROUPS

**Proteins.** Proteins are very important at this time to keep your child's digestion warm, promote growth, and boost immunity. You can smash meat and serve it next to a side of veggies. Having some kind of meat for lunch and dinner meal should provide your child with adequate protein intake.

**Dairy.** Introduce dairy slowly as it may cause allergies. Only give one form of dairy (besides formula or breast milk) per day, and start with yogurt or a soft cheese. You may introduce milk alternatives at this time, such as oat milk or almond milk. Generally, avoid soymilk because soy is really cold to the digestion, which may interfere with your child's maturing digestive system.

**Pasta.** Try to give your growing child pasta-based foods no more than three times a week to avoid allergies and blood sugar problems. Wheat-based foods may slow the digestive system and cause phlegm build-up and mucous-related illnesses.

**Nuts.** Try to avoid peanut butter as long as possible. Peanut butter may have aflatoxins and sometimes molds. This leads to allergies, phlegm, and liver congestion. Alternatives are tahini, sunflower butter, almond butter, etc.

**Honey.** It is still considered prudent to avoid raw honey until your child is one years old. Honey can contain spores of a bacterium called *Clostridium botulinum*, which can germinate in a baby's immature digestive system and cause infant botulism, a rare but potentially fatal illness. These spores are usually harmless to adults and children over one years old because the microorganisms normally found in the intestine keep the bacteria from growing. (Mayo Clinic, 2018)

## ■ STAYING HYDRATED

As you're decreasing the number of bottles your baby is taking, remember to keep your child very hydrated. The first beverage choice should be water to help develop taste in the sense you're not starting with something sweet. Try natural lemonade if you want to give some juice. Lemonade is not as cold for the digestion as other juices and doesn't cause blood sugar fluctuations like other fruit juices. It's also nice to add a sour taste to a mostly sweet and bland diet. If you do give other kinds of juice, consider it your one piece of fruit for the day. At the end of the day, it is best to wait until after 12 months for any juice.

You may begin to give your child solid food at snack times, to begin to replace breast milk or formula by 18 months.

## ■ EXPAND BABY'S FOOD TEXTURES

Some children are very sensitive to the texture of food, but if you can offer foods in a variety of textures at an early age, your baby may develop a broader palette for food that he is willing to eat.

You may start baby off with very smooth purees, but every few weeks, increase the "chunkiness" of the food that you're offering. Eventually, you want baby to explore chewing soft food. Once she has more teeth, she might enjoy soft but firm food, and eventually even crisp or crunchy food. Be aware of the variety of textures you're offering her.

# BABY'S SECOND YEAR AND BEYOND

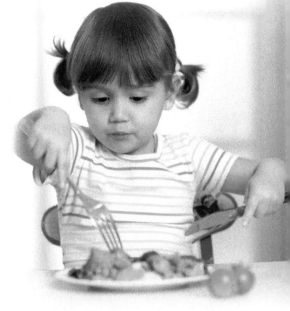

As your child begins to interact with more children and environments, her immune system will become important to you and your family. Little children are exposed to so many viruses and bacteria, but if they have resilient health, they will be able to avoid prolonged illnesses, and you will be spared a constantly sick household!

Resilient health begins with effective digestion. Focusing on warm foods, meats, vegetables, and occasional fruit and grains will help your baby develop, and keep, a digestive system that will promote a strong immune system.

Adhering to the principles in this book is especially important when your child is:

1.  teething

2.  sick

3.  going through a growth spurt or developmental milestone

4.  receiving vaccinations

5.  in an unusual environment

6.  exposed to viruses, bacteria, and allergens

## ■ IN TIMES OF CHANGE AND SICKNESS

Just because your child is not hungry does not mean that he is sick. Infants and children usually have reduced appetites during teething and developmental growth periods. As long as he is not showing a fever, vomiting, or other health concerns that your pediatrician has indicated as a problematic symptom, his appetite may return to normal within a few days. If a regular appetite does not return with the resolution of the illness, check with your pediatrician.

But, also note that not all illnesses are bad! Remember, every three to six months, your child may go through "changing syndromes" or "steaming syndromes," manifested with phlegm and a warmer body temperature, but these syndromes typically precede growth and development milestones and should pass fairly quickly.

If you notice consistent phlegm or constipation, you should revisit the principles we've discussed in this book, and work with a healthcare provider to prevent and recover from illnesses.

# TO SUM UP

It can be unnerving to introduce new foods to your baby's digestive system, but if you are intentional and methodical about what foods you offer your little one, you can set your child up for good nutritional habits that will last her a lifetime. These are the years when her preferences are developing and she's most open to new tastes and textures. If she learns to eat healthy, warm foods now, she can prevent illness, pains, and allergies for years to come, without as much effort, as her habits will already be established.

It's important to remember that when your baby is sick, in pain, or stressed, that causes you a lot of worry and heartache. In the end…

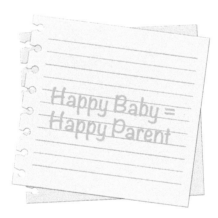

You may feel like you can't feed your baby a perfect diet every day, and that's okay, but the more you can incorporate these principles into your baby's nutrition, the happier and healthier you and your whole family will be.

# ABOUT THE AUTHOR

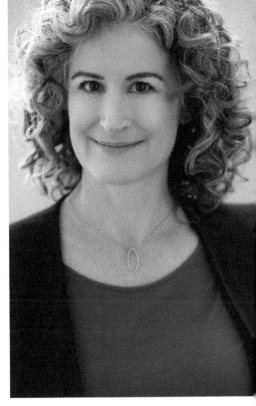

Tansy Briggs is an Integrative Acupuncture and Chinese Medicine Practitioner.

She is passionate about educating as many people as possible about how the balance of good nutrition and keeping their digestion warm can transform their health!

Tansy Briggs, DACM, Dipl. O.M. (NCCAOM), and Licensed Acupuncturist, is an Integrative Acupuncture and Chinese Medicine Practitioner. Her licenses, certificates, and diplomas include: nationally board certified as a Diplomate in Oriental Medicine (Dipl. O.M.) by the NCCAOM (National Certification Commission for Acupuncture and Oriental Medicine), a Licensed Practitioner of Oriental Medicine (L.OM) in Pennsylvania and Licensed Acupuncturist (L.Ac) in Colorado. Tansy completed her Doctor of Acupuncture and Chinese Medicine (DACM) with Pacific College of Oriental Medicine, San Diego in 2018 and obtained her Master of Science in Oriental Medicine (MSOM) from Southwest Acupuncture College in 2001 in Santa Fe, NM. Prior to acupuncture college, Tansy studied natural medicine for three years in Santa Fe via seminars and mentorships. Her bachelor's degree is from Clark University in Worcester, MA. Prior to graduation, Tansy spent her last undergraduate year abroad at the University of East Anglia, UK. You can learn more about Tansy Briggs at www. tansybriggs.com.

# ADDITIONAL RESOURCES

Books

*The Key to A Healthy Digestion: How To Eat Warm and Cold Foods To Improve Your Health* by Tansy Briggs

*Healing with Whole Foods: Asian Traditions and Modern Nutrition (3rd edition)* by Paul Pitchford

*Chinese Pediatric Massage Therapy: A Parent's and Practitioner's Guide to the Treatment and Prevention of Childhood Diseases* by Fan Ya-Li

*Keeping Your Child Healthy with Chinese Medicine: A Parent's Guide to the Care and Prevention of Common Childhood Diseases* by Bob Flaws

*7 Times a Woman: Ancient Wisdom on Health & Beauty for Every Stage of Your Life* by Dr. Lia Andrews

# WORKS CITED

American Academy of Pediatrics. (2017, May 22) AAP.org. "American Academy of Pediatrics Recommends No Fruit Juice For Children Under 1 Year." Retrieved August 2, 2019 from https://www.aap.org/en-us/about-the-aap/aap-press-room/Pages/American-Academy-of-Pediatrics-Recommends-No-Fruit-Juice-For-Children-Under-1-Year.aspx.

American Academy of Pediatrics. (2015, Dec 8) HealthyChildren.org. Retrieved August 2, 2019 from https://www.healthychildren.org/English/ages-stages/baby/feeding-nutrition/Pages/Sample-One-Day-Menu-for-an-8-to-12-Month-Old.aspx.

Bhutta, Z. A. (2013, March 28) "Early Nutrition and Adult Outcomes: Pieces of the Puzzle." *The Lancet.*

Harvard Medical School. (2017, Sept 20) Harvard Health Publishing. "Microwaving Food in Plastic: Dangerous or Not?" Retrieved August 2, 2019 from health.harvard.edu: https://www.health.harvard.edu/staying-healthy/microwaving-food-in-plastic-dangerous-or-not.

Institute of Medicine. (1991) *Nutrition During Lactation.* "Meeting Maternal Nutrient Needs During Lactation." Washington, DC: National Academies Press.

Mayo Clinic. (2018, May 15) MayoClinic.org. "How Can I Protect My Baby from Infant Botulism?" Retrieved August 2, 2019 from https://www.mayoclinic.org/healthy-lifestyle/infant-and-toddler-health/expert-answers/infant-botulism/faq-20058477.

Mohrbacher, N. (2019) "Diaper Output and Milk Intake in the Early Weeks." Retrieved August 2, 2019 from https://breastfeedingusa.org/content/article/diaper-output-and-milk-intake-early-weeks.

CPSIA information can be obtained
at www.ICGtesting.com
Printed in the USA
LVHW070812280720
661671LV00028B/350/J